LIVING WITH PANCREATIC CANCER

My Experience as a Carer

Ann Elizabeth Bruce

All Rights Reserved

Copyright Ann Elizabeth Bruce 2013

No part of this book may be reproduced in any form by photocopying or by any electronic or mechanical means, including information storage and retrieval systems, without permission in writing from both the copyright owner and the publisher of this book.

This book is sold subject to the condition that it shall not, by way of trade or otherwise, be lent, resold, hired out, or otherwise circulated in any form of binding or cover other than that in which it is published.

INTRODUCTION

I am writing this book, using my online blog diary as reference. http://livingwithpancreaticcancer.blogspot.co.uk/ I wrote the blog diary during the course of 2012 whilst caring for my close friend and companion Margaret. It was written as it happened. Although using the original entries there are events and incidents that have been triggered by going back over the blog pages, these are also included in the book. I'm hoping my experiences both physical and emotional, might help others going through a similar situation, not necessarily Pancreatic Cancer, but caring for someone with a terminal illness.

My life was changed forever from the moment my friend was admitted to hospital, on 8th May 2012 to the present.

My intention is to tell it how it was, honestly and sometimes with raw emotion.

I hope you will find it of help whatever your circumstances.

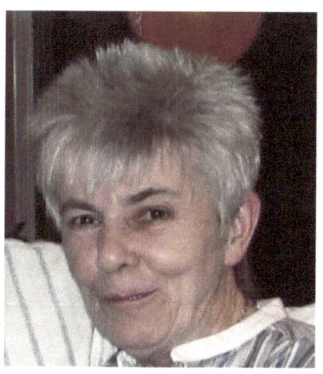

MARGARET

1st April 1945 – 13th November 2012

HOW IT ALL BEGAN

The year of 2012 was a perfectly normal year, whatever normal is! It was the year of the Olympics being held in Great Britain and the celebration of the Queen's Jubilee. Much to look forward to you would think, but for me it was a year that I would rather forget but never will.

I shared my house with Margaret as I had for some 10 years. For some months she had been complaining of severe stomach pains. They were usually most severe at night, which I later found out was part of the symptoms of pancreatic cancer as the pain is always more severe whilst lying down. She had also complained of constant itching and couldn't stop scratching, making herself sore in places. Again this was another symptom. Toxins were trying to escape through the skin, because the pancreas was blocked and could not do its work properly. But again these symptoms were ignored and put down to a change in washing detergent.

Because Margaret had a history of stomach problems having had a major operation on her stomach in her 20's, she assumed that it was connected in some way and therefore did not consult her G.P. for some time, as her opinion of the doctors at the local surgery was considerably negative.

I did have a conversation with her about her reasons for not going to the G.P., it went something like this:-

'Are you frightened of going to the doctor in case they say it is cancer' – Me

'It probably is, but no I'm not frightened.' – Margaret.

'Then why don't you go?' – Me

'You know how useless they are' – Margaret.

And there ended the conversation.

However eventually the pains became so unbearable that Margaret made an appointment. She said that she could feel a lump in her stomach. I had a feel and there was definitely something unusual, but I said that I couldn't feel anything, because I thought if I said I could feel something she would get really worried.

The appointment made, the visit to the doctor just exacerbated the situation. He also assumed that the pains were associated with her previous medical history and said that he couldn't feel a lump, even though Margaret showed him the exact spot. Needless to say I don't think Margaret mentioned the itching. I can't say for sure because at this stage, Margaret wouldn't allow me to go with her to see the doctor. Because of his assumption he prescribed some medication. Within 24 hours she came up in a rash and was extremely ill. She was allergic to the medication. Her urine went dark brown and her skin (to me at least) began to look yellow, She couldn't see it and said that it was her natural skin colour.

Because she was so poorly, I helped her to the bathroom and was quite shocked when she undressed to see how thin she had become. I had lived with her 24 hours a day and hadn't noticed, but I never saw her without clothes. She was either dressed or in her PJ's. How could I have missed it. I didn't say anything, but hoped that my face hadn't given anything away.

A few days later a return visit was made to the doctors surgery. I could see that her skin was yellow, but the whites of her eyes were not affected. She saw the Practice Nurse as there wasn't an appointment available with a doctor. Now if I could see that Margaret was yellow how come the Practice Nurse failed to notice. Instead she asked Margaret to give a urine sample. Her diagnosis was a urine infection and an allergy surprise, surprise. Margaret was given antibiotics for the urine infection and antihistamine for the rash.

Over the next five days (it was the May Bank Holiday weekend) Margaret took her medication. Now whilst the antihistamine did help the rash, the antibiotics did nothing for the 'urine infection' .Well I never. She was becoming more and more jaundiced despite her self denial of the fact.

Finally on the Tuesday after the Bank Holiday, Margaret saw herself in the mirror, the whites of her eyes were now yellow, so she could finally see it for herself. Confirmation from the visiting hairdresser, who as soon as she walked through the door remarked on how yellow Margaret looked, spurred her to make an emergency appointment with the doctor.

At 4.20 pm Tuesday 8th May 2012 the relief doctor on duty told Margaret that she must go straight to hospital because she was seriously ill. She had gone in to see him on her own, but soon came out to fetch me when she realised how serious it was. From that point on I always attended the appointments with her. She wasn't going to go to the hospital, but the doctor persuaded her by saying it was only for some tests, because he thought it might be cancer, but she would be coming home again after the tests. He lied! This was the moment that not only changed my friends life, but also my own.

THE FIRST HOSPITAL VISIT

Before we traveled to the hospital, we went back home to give our dogs their tea. Anything to delay the inevitable. We always took the dogs everywhere with us, so Margaret was insistent that they came with us to the hospital. I disagreed and said it was silly to do so, knowing deep down that she would be kept in. However the dogs came.

The 26 mile journey to the nearest hospital with an on call doctor versed in such matters as jaundice was fraught with tension. Margaret was petrified and determined not to be admitted, smoking, (yes she was still smoking), more cigarettes than she should. Those cigarettes she smoked on that tense journey were to be her last. From that day until the day she passed, she never smoked again. She did say some weeks later,
'I don't know why I haven't stopped before because I haven't missed not smoking'

But I think her body had made the decision for her, because she had smoked since she was 11 years old and had always said,
'I've smoked since I was eleven and it's never done me any harm, I haven't even got a cough'.

How wrong she was. On arrival at the hospital we were to report to the Accident and Emergency department and give in a quickly hand written letter by the G.P. outlining the problem.

When we arrived the first problem was finding a parking space in the shade for the dogs, as it turned out to be a very warm sunny evening. By now the time was about 6.30 pm. The parking space secured we made our way to A & E. The place was packed. Having been assured by the G.P. that we would not have to wait once we were booked in, imagine our horror when we were told to take a seat. However the G.P was right, within about 10 minutes we were called through to a cubicle.

The consultant immediately began to take a history and took blood samples. Margaret was shocked when the consultant said that she would have to stay in for further tests. She argued the point quite vigorously, but he was insistent that she was going to be admitted and I think then she realized that she had no choice. She was very upset and began to cry. I was at sixes and sevens because we hadn't prepared for this, in as much as I had gone along with her belief that she would not be kept in. Because she believed what the G.P. had told her, we had taken nothing with us, no PJ's or toiletries, so it looked like a hospital gown was the garment of choice for the first night at least.

I waited with my friend for what seemed like ages. There were no vacant beds immediately and the consultant wasn't sure when one would become available. Margaret began to stress because of the dogs still waiting in the car. I must admit I did feel like saying 'I told you so', but resisted the temptation as I didn't feel it was appropriate or would solve anything. She was also getting stressed because she didn't want me driving home in the middle of the night. So she insisted I went home, with a list of what to bring the following day. Again not being prepared all I could find was a scrap of paper in my bag. When I got home I couldn't understand half of what I had written.

After some heated words about not leaving her to go through these tests alone and the dogs would be fine for a little longer, I regrettably left Margaret to fend for herself and to wait for a vacant bed. She never knew, but I was extremely upset having to leave her in such circumstances. I know I would have wanted someone with me if I was in the same position. Yet there was part of me that was relieved that I didn't have to stay. But then that gave me feelings of guilt that I should even consider being relieved. I hate hospitals even for visiting.

When I reached the car the dogs were all excited and I did my best to explain to them what had happened through streams of tears and heaving sobs. I must admit they were very good, they didn't make a fuss and seemed to understand. I eventually managed to stop crying and drove home. The house seemed very empty. Little did I know then what lie ahead and how lonely I would feel a year later.

At 10 pm that evening I telephoned the hospital and was put through to the ward where Margaret had finally been found a bed. I was told that albeit reluctantly she had settled in and was hooked up to a saline drip.

What happened over the next few weeks can only be described as the most mind blowing, shocking and devastating news that can be given to anyone.

THE FIRST EIGHT DAYS IN HOSPITAL

For the next eight days Margaret was put through various tests to ascertain what was causing the jaundice. She had x-rays, ultra sound and CT scans. Her fluid intake and output were monitored for fear of kidney failure. She had a chart where she had to mark down how many fluid ounces she drank. She then had to pee in a special cardboard urine container so that the nurses could measure what was coming out. Despite all the tests and the fear of kidney failure and still being bright yellow, she seemed to remain relatively well, although desperate to get home.

She was so well in fact that she was showering unsupervised and still eating small amounts. The nurses allowed her to walk down to the hospital shop and get a newspaper each day and we met in the hospital coffee shop each afternoon, so allowing more visiting time. Instead of having to wait until 2.30 pm we could meet earlier at 2 pm and then go back on to the ward later for me to pick up the dirty washing, drop off clean PJ's and anything else that she had requested.

I must admit the 26 mile trip to and from the hospital each day was tiring and the whole day had to be geared around the visit. The dogs had to be left for a few hours each day, something they hadn't been use to as there was always someone at home, but they adapted very well and didn't seem too concerned about Margaret's absence.

When not at the hospital I began to research Margaret's symptoms and it soon became all to apparent that she had pancreatic cancer, it really didn't need a consultant to tell me that. All the signs had been there but of course were ignored. I must admit at the time I questioned myself as to whether I should have been more forceful and made her go to the doctor. Would it have made any difference? It is something I shall never know. I do believe that when it is our time to die nothing in this world will change it. On one of my many visits to the hospital I did discuss with Margaret what I had found on the internet. She didn't seem surprised!

After 7 days I was summoned to a meeting with the registrar, a specialist nurse and a ward nurse to discuss what had been found. Initially the registrar was cagey, wouldn't commit himself, but in the end admitted that he was 95% sure that it was pancreatic cancer., but wouldn't be 100% sure until an Endoscopy was carried out. He did say that it was a fairly large tumour.

This of course wasn't a shock as we had already discussed the diagnosis of pancreatic cancer from my own extensive research. So what next. A permanent drain would be fitted in order to remove the excess bile causing the jaundice. This would also continue to remove the bile so that the jaundice would not return. It would only be when this was fitted that Margaret would be allowed home. It was felt that this was the best place for her as she would be more content and secure.

Well I'm not sure how Margaret coped with the operation to fit the drain. She hated anaesthetics and even local anaesthetics took ages to work. A visit to the dentist requiring an injection was pointless because it wasn't until she returned home that it began to work. Anyway I digress. She said that she thought she was going to die as the drain was fitted, but somehow she coped. The drain was accompanied by a very unattractive bag, not the best designer wear. It had to be carried over the shoulder, It had a drain on the bottom which had to be empted down the toilet when full, but by the time it was full it was so heavy that it had to be emptied far more often. Because she had to wear the bag 24/7 I had to rig up a hook on the bedside table so that at night she could hang the bag on the hook.

Within 24 hours of the drain being fitted, Margaret returned home, to await the Endoscopy appointment. She wasn't given any medication as it was felt she didn't need it at that time, but in hindsight I think they were wrong as I found out a few weeks later at a time when I couldn't contact anyone. The fact that she was home made her feel 100 times better., especially now in familiar surroundings. It was for me a worrying time as I now had the responsibility of caring for her, which was quite a daunting task. She never was a good patient so the road was going to be rocky.

It was arranged for a district nurse to come in to take bloods and to check the dressing and the wound where the drain had been fitted. It couldn't have been at all comfortable. The area surrounding the tube where it entered the body looked very sore and was obviously distressing. But Margaret never made a fuss. She just seemed to accept it.

It was strange really because we never really discussed what

Margaret had been through, how she felt, how I felt, we just seemed to get on with it. The only conversation about the future happened a couple of days after she returned home and it went like this'

'What will you do when I'm not here?' – Margaret.

'I really don't know, I haven't thought about it. I might stay here, I might move, I really don't know' – Me.

'Will you keep the dogs?' – Margaret.

'Of course I will, there is no question about that' – Me.

'I want a civil funeral, no hymns and I want my ashes to be put in the front garden' –Margaret.

'OK' –Me.

We never talked about it again.

THE ENDOSCOPY

A phone call received a few days after she returned home confirmed an appointment for an Endoscopy. This was booked for Monday 28th May at 9.30 am. Unfortunately the Endoscopy was to be carried out in a hospital in the next county. So not only was Margaret having to put up with all the discomfort, she now had to be up, washed, dressed and ready to leave home at 8 am. No mean task under the circumstances. We arranged a car through NHS transport as this seemed the easiest way to get her there on time as they knew where to go. Margaret was yet again stressed about leaving the dogs for a long time at home. She wouldn't let me take her as it was assumed that she would be all day. She insisted that I stayed with the dogs.

I didn't like the idea of Margaret going for something so major as this with a complete stranger, but I knew to argue would be futile and would only stress her even more than she already was. So I gave in gracefully and sat and worried about her at home. As it happened it was a very friendly lady who came for Margaret, who put her at ease straight away, so I wasn't quite so concerned.

As always Margaret refused any sedative for the procedure, because she didn't want to spend a moment longer in the hospital than she had to. I'm not sure whether it was a brave or stupid thing to do, but if she had a sedative she would have to wait at least 2 hours after the procedure before she would have been allowed home. I know I certainly couldn't have swallowed a large black tube with a camera on the end without some sort of help. It also transpired that the NHS transport car was on a limited time for the return journey, so I think that clinched the deal so to speak.

The experience was very painful and Margaret thought she was definitely dying, even more so than the drain operation. She said that she couldn't breathe and it felt like her chest was going to burst. The only thing that kept her going was the thought of getting home quickly. Whilst the procedure was being carried out a small biopsy was meant to be taken. However this was overlooked and whilst Margaret was recovering in the waiting room the technician came in and said that he hadn't read the form properly and hadn't taken the biopsy and would Margaret wait and have it done again. Well I think by now you can imagine the response. Needless to say she didn't have the procedure again. In hindsight, I guess we should have put in a complaint, but with everything else to cope with, it never happened.

As it happened she arrived back home just before lunch time, so I could have taken her, the dogs would have been fine. The only thing now was to wait for the result. We didn't have to wait long. The following day we received a phone call from the hospital where Margaret had the Endoscopy. It was from a nurse talking about operations and all sorts. A very frightening conversation and not one I think should have been carried out over the phone.

A few hours later Margaret received another phone call from the local hospital 26 miles away to say that she had been slotted in for an appointment on Thursday 31st May at 10.10 am with the *consultant surgeon. Now she would really find out what was going to happen.*

THE CONSULTANT MEETING

We arrived at the hospital in good time, albeit it had been a rush to get Margaret washed, dressed and ready. As well as walking the dogs, feeding them and getting myself washed, breakfasted and ready. But we made it. We made our way to the outpatient clinic only to find that they were already running 30 minutes late, so we knew we would have a wait. What a pain, you then start thinking, I needn't have rushed. Around 50 minutes later we were called in to see the consultant.

He was very pleasant and frank about Margaret's situation. He confirmed that she had indeed got pancreatic cancer and the prognosis as it stood was 6-18 months. A mind blowing and devastating statement. He then went on to explain the possible options.

Although the growth was 4 cm in diameter, which normally wouldn't be considered for an operation, he felt that the pictures from the scans and the results of the endoscopy indicated that removal was a possibility, but confirmation of this would not be possible until they opened her up. Even then removal may not mean a cure and even if an immediate cure could be achieved the growth would be likely to come back in a few years.

The second option would be re-constructive surgery, which would mean creating a bypass around the growth. This would negate the need for the drain and bag and would alleviate symptoms, such as sickness and being unable to eat. This could either be carried out as a separate operation or if unable to remove the growth once opened up.

The third option was a procedure under sedation which would allow the removal of the drain and bag, but would still mean having the bypass operation, but this could happen at a later date.

This was a huge amount of information to take on board and make a decision about. So Margaret was given 7 days to think about it and a return appointment was made for 6th June at 10 am.

THE NEXT SEVEN DAYS

Not only had my friend to think about her options, but suddenly her general health and day to day struggle with what had now been confirmed as a fatal disease was becoming increasingly difficult.

Up until this point I had helped Margaret to dress and maintained the day to day running of the home. Cleaning, cooking, walking the dogs etc. But suddenly she took a dramatic turn for the worse. She was now unable to stand or walk for more than a few seconds. It was so sudden. One day she could do most things for herself with minimum assistance, the next I find I'm having to do everything for her. Washing her, drying her, everything to do with her personal care.

What little food she had been eating, now dropped to nearly nothing. The amount she was managing to consume wouldn't have kept a baby alive. She was still drinking, but only small amounts. She was in constant discomfort, but not what could be classed as real pain.

Over the next few days Margaret got steadily worse. It didn't help that it was the Queen's Jubilee extended weekend, making it 4 days without being able to contact anyone for advice as everyone was on holiday. The last contact with anyone was with the district nurse on the Thursday before the Bank Holiday weekend began. Apart from that we hadn't had any support.

The appointment at the hospital to decide how to move forward was looking increasingly less likely. It would need an overnight miracle.

THE CRISIS

By the Tuesday afternoon, things got even worse. Margaret began vomiting and continued overnight and into the next morning. She got to the stage where she couldn't even keep fluids down so was becoming dehydrated. Her bones were protruding through her skin, the deterioration had been very dramatic.

I was beside myself with worry. I wanted to call the emergency services, but even in her dreadful state Margaret would have none of it. She didn't want to have to go through the whole process of explaining everything, she just wanted to speak to someone who knew what they were talking about. I must admit I did lose it a bit that weekend. I ended up shouting at her,
'How the hell can I help you if you won't let me, you're so bloody stubborn, this is never going to work unless you help me'.
It didn't make a blind bit of difference.

On the Wednesday morning 6th June, the day of the consultant appointment, I was on the phone. It wasn't even 7 am. I left messages on answer phones, everywhere I could think of. District nurses office, the specialist nurses office, just anyone I thought might listen. At around 8.30 am the specialist nurse phoned from the hospital. I told her the problem and at first she suggested going to the G.P. Well I'm sorry, if she thought I was going to try and get Margaret to the G.P. who up until this point had not seen her since the initial appointment on the 8th May, then she could think again. She got the message and after some phone calls to the consultant called me back to say that Margaret would be re-admitted as soon as they found a bed, which may take some hours.

Waiting for the phone call to say a bed had been found seemed like days. All the while Margaret was still vomiting and sinking fast. I must admit I thought then that it was the end. If I didn't get her to hospital soon she wouldn't be alive to take the bed. Finally at 2 pm the phone rang. At last a bed had been found. We could have waited for an ambulance, but that was going to add yet more hours onto Margaret's already dehydrated, exhausted body. I said I would bring her in the car.

THE SECOND STAY IN HOSPITAL

I wrapped Margaret in a fleece dressing gown over her PJ's, found an old bowl as she was still vomiting although very little was actually coming out. I'd already packed her bag. We were off. The journey was difficult. Trying to keep an eye on Margaret and watch to road. I pulled up outside the main entrance to the hospital, grabbed a wheelchair and got her into it. I then had to abandon her whilst I went and parked the car. We made it onto the ward by 2.45 pm. She was put in a side room and immediately hooked up to a drip and various drugs were pumped into her to ease the pain and stop her vomiting. All I could do now was wait and hope that the treatment worked. Being put in a side room, unless you're paying for it is always a bit ominous!

I went home thinking I would get a phone call from the hospital during the night to say it was all over, she was really that bad, but none was received. The following day 7th June I spoke to her on the phone and she sounded much better. The medication was obviously working. I would be seeing her later so hopefully I would find out much more.

I didn't find out very much on my visit, but she was looking a lot better. The medication had kicked in and she was now starting to eat and drink again. Very small amounts of what she fancied.

On 8th June she saw the consultant and he told her that it was up to her if she wanted to go home. But still not feeling well she opted to stay in the hospital, so I knew just how ill she was because she wouldn't make a decision like that lightly. She was told that no operations were going to take place at that time.

Now something I must just mention here. The staff at the hospital were all wonderful, neither Margaret or myself could fault their care and understanding apart from one who really upset Margaret by saying and I quote,

'You can't spend the rest of your time in a hospital bed and you should go home'.

Again we should have complained but didn't as we had too much else to contend with. Margaret felt awful, it really got to her and she did speak to another nurse about it, who was very sympathetic, but I don't think anything was done.

On the morning of Saturday 9th June a registrar paid Margaret a visit. He confirmed that she would not be allowed home until a good support network was in place. Monday was a possibility, but it would depend on the support network. She managed a shower on her own although it took her over an hour with many periods of sitting down. Walking was now more of a problem she was only able to walk extremely short distances before needing to sit down with exhaustion. She found this extremely frustrating and became very upset. She was a very active person always doing and found this restriction difficult to take on board. She was definitely in a better place than the previous weekend, but still had a very long way to go.

She spent a fairly good weekend in hospital. On Monday 11th June she was told that she was to undergo an operation on the Thursday. This was going to be under local anaesthetic. A titanium stent was to be fitted to replace the external drain and bag. She was not looking forward to that. In view of that the earliest she was going to *be home was Friday, dependent on how she was feeling. Chemotherapy was now being mentioned, but a major operation was now definitely not on the cards.*

ARRIVAL OF EQUIPMENT

In the meantime back at home, the district nurses had been busy ordering equipment for Margaret's return. A special mattress to stop pressure sores/bed sores, a pillow lift/backrest for the bed and a cushion for use in the wheelchair that had also been ordered.

Well on the morning of the 12th June they arrived. They were huge. The pillow/lift/back rest which could be raised or lowered remotely once plugged into the mains, weighed an absolute ton and took up half the length of the bed. This in turn was to sit on top of the 6 inch thick mattress covered in plastic in case of accidents so that it could be wiped clean. I was unsure as to where exactly Margaret was meant to sleep and she would have needed a ladder to get into bed.

Whoever designed these things obviously had no idea as to the size of normal household furniture. There was no way that we would be using the equipment and I stored it very carefully in the garage until such times as I could return it. The wheelchair cushion was also useless. When the wheelchair arrived a few days later it had its own cushion. So this was also stored and returned. I know they meant well, but it was just something else to worry about.

THE OPERATION AND COMING HOME

Margaret had her operation under sedation, although she said that as usual it didn't really do anything and she felt it all. It was rather painful, but a small price to pay to be rid of 'Dolly' the name she had given her drainage bag. Apparently the titanium stent was massive in length and she couldn't believe that all of it was going inside her, but it did.

She was given a small temporary drain just in case the stent didn't work. Providing all was OK this part was to be removed on the Saturday morning the 16th June and then all being well should would be allowed home. She was ecstatic at the prospect of coming home.

She now had to carry a card to say that she had a titanium tube inside her, just in case anything went wrong. We hoped it wouldn't and it never did.

Margaret was given a date for an appointment with the Oncologist for 21st June at 3.30 pm. This is to discuss the possibility of Chemotherapy.

On 16th June Margaret was sent home. This time she was given loads of medication for pain and stopping the sickness., so we should be covered for every eventuality. For someone who hated even taking a paracetamol for a headache, she had so many pills to take I thought I was going to have problems getting her to take them, but she never complained and just took them when she was given them. I knew she was really suffering because that just wasn't Margaret, she would have sooner died (excuse the pun) than take a tablet. So not only was I her carer, I was now her pharmacist too.

She had good and bad days and her eating wasn't very good. I suppose at least she was eating something. It was a right pain I can tell you, trying to find things that she would eat. The district nurse had bought in a load of those high calorie, drinks and yoghurts, which were on prescription. Margaret had already said that she didn't want them as she had tried them whilst in hospital and hated them. But the district nurse hadn't listened. When the district nurse arrived with them Margaret repeated this but the nurse was insistent that she tried them. After she had left Margaret wasn't very pleasant about the poor nurse, who after all was only trying to do her job. The drinks and yoghurts ended up in a cupboard and eventually I took them back to the pharmacy.

So trying to find foods Margaret would eat was a nightmare. I would find something that she would eat, so bought a few more, only to be stuck with them because she never ate it again. I became extremely frustrated by this, but getting annoyed with her about it only made things worse. She refused to eat anything.

I was still having to do everything for her, although she was managing to shower herself as we had been provided with a shower seat. An absolute Godsend, without it I'm not sure how I would have managed. I still hovered outside the shower to make sure she was OK and I still had to help her with drying and dressing.

Because she was now so thin, I also had to check for any signs of pressure sores. I creamed the areas most vulnerable with body lotion as her skin was becoming very dry. This became a daily routine. Instead of the monstrous mattress, I invested in a memory foam mattress topper, which did the trick and was far less cumbersome.

CHEMOTHERAPY

At 3.30 pm on 21st June we went for the appointment with the Oncologist, to the local hospital 26 miles away where Margaret had spent time as an inpatient. He told Margaret that in his opinion she had made the right decision by not having the operation to remove the tumour, as the probability was that once opened up it wouldn't be suitable for removal anyway. He continued by saying that even though she hadn't had the biopsy, from the results he had seen he was quite happy to proceed with Chemotherapy, if that was what Margaret wanted, as he was 99.99% certain that it was Pancreatic Cancer.

On the 25th June we made the journey yet again to the local hospital to see the Chemotherapy suite, meet the nurses and get a feel for the place. Margaret was given times and dates for her treatments. She was also told by the Specialist Nurse that even with chemotherapy treatment, she could only expect a couple of months extension to her life.

At the time I didn't think that I would put myself through all that just for a couple of months and now a year later I still feel the same. More so now as I know what happened which at the time I didn't. At that time I thought that you didn't really know how you would react until it happened to you. But whatever my feelings on the subject I thought Margaret was very brave to even consider it, let alone go through with it.

The chemotherapy treatment began on Friday 29th June. The treatment itself took about half an hour, but there were certain procedures that needed to be carried out before and after the treatment, making the whole process an hour. That in itself seemed fine, until you realised that you didn't always get in on time, because there had been problems with previous patients and a suitable vein wasn't always easy to find. So often the procedure took much longer than an hour.

Once a suitable vein was found and a cannula was fitted, the first process was a flush through with saline, then the chemotherapy was attached and various pills were taken to stop sickness, then once the chemotherapy had gone through then another period of flush through with saline. At any one time there were probably 10 patients on the go with various types of chemotherapy. All had to be double checked by two members of staff to make sure the right one was being given to the right person. So even when the time was up, Margaret still had to sometimes wait to be unhooked.

As well as the tablets to stop the sickness, the particular chemotherapy that Margaret was being given, could cause blood clots so she needed a daily injection of 'Clexane' a blood thinning drug, in her stomach. This was to be given by the District Nurses. However we never knew when they were going to arrive, as they had other more urgent patients to attend. It could have been self administered but Margaret didn't feel she would be able to do that, but was happy for me to do it. So after a couple of days I asked if they would show me how to do it, then I could give her the injection at our convenience. They agreed. They would still need to come every Thursday to take bloods for the chemotherapy on Friday, but at least it was only one day.

Every day for 3 months I injected Margaret in the stomach. As time went on it became increasingly more difficult to find enough flesh. I had to make sure that it wasn't too near her belly button and scar from her operation in her 20's, squeeze a portion of flesh between my finger and thumb and then inject. I had to build myself up to it every day because I knew it was painful. At this point more than anything I'd done before I was now treating Margaret as a patient not my friend and companion. I had stepped back from our relationship completely. I had to otherwise I don't think I would have coped with it all.

The chemotherapy was once a week for 7 weeks, then a weeks break. The treatment would then re-start, the frequency at this stage was still to be decided.

After 2 weeks of chemotherapy the side effects hadn't been as bad as anticipated. Margaret often felt nauseous for the first couple of days, but was never physically sick and was fortunate not to get the other adverse side effect of the runs, which knowing her previous history was a miracle. The fact was that if anything she was constipated and yet more medication was required to alleviate the problem.

Eating was becoming a problem again as everything she ate she said tasted horrible. It was the chemotherapy causing the funny taste in her mouth, but that was of no help when eating was a problem anyway. The other concern was that she had no energy, which was not really surprising, but she was now spending far more time in bed.

However overall we didn't grumble. We were still ploughing on taking each day, if not each moment as it came. Chemotherapy continued and by Friday 20th July it was her forth session, which unfortunately didn't take place as her blood count was too low. But we didn't find this out until we got to the hospital so had a wasted journey. But it would at least give her body a rest and time to recover. She still felt very nauseous, not just for a couple of days, but on an off throughout the week. She remained very weak and was spending more and more time in bed.

I couldn't see how the chemotherapy was achieving anything. All I saw was my friend and companion getting thinner and thinner, eating less and less and becoming weaker and weaker. I couldn't see how it was or how it would improve her quality of life. But then who was I? I wasn't a doctor, just her carer who spent 24 hours a day with her. I just saw her getting worse and wondered if she would have been any different or better had she not agreed to have the chemotherapy.

It was her decision to try the chemotherapy and it was her decision when to stop it. Whatever she decided and how ever long she had on the earth plain, I was going to stand by her.

On 24th July we attended a clinic. Margaret was weighed and she had lost another 6.6 kg roughly 12 lb. It wasn't any wonder she was looking so thin. She was put back on some medication she had taken before, which would hopefully improve her appetite. The combination of medication and a break from chemotherapy saw a little improvement.

Chemotherapy took place on Friday 27th July. This was one of the days where we had to wait for ages before the treatment began, because earlier in the day the computers had crashed and put everything behind as the blood results etc. couldn't be accessed. It was very frustrating but there was nothing we could do to change it, so just had to grin and bear it.

AT LAST SOME IMPROVEMENT

Unusually Margaret, felt much better after her chemotherapy and an added bonus was that she had started to fancy food. Some of it was a little strange but that didn't matter, she was eating more than she had for weeks. They were still not normal size portions but it was at least normal food.

She fancied fish finger sandwiches, pate on oatmeal biscuits, poached egg on toast, chicken and roast potatoes, ham, new potatoes and beetroot. The portions were only enough to fit on a tea plate, but it was far superior to mousse or a cup of noodle soup, minus the noodles.

On 30th July we managed a trip to the supermarket. I pushed Margaret in her wheelchair, she took control of the basket. This was a triumph. For weeks now I had dashed to the supermarket on my own or bought from the village mini market, so to actually be able to take a fairly leisurely trip to the local supermarket was a delight. Unfortunately the following day the 31st July, Margaret had a setback, having a lot of pain. After some medication it passed. Whatever happened it was not over we would keep fighting.

Two more weeks of chemotherapy and things continued to improve, especially eating. She was now fancying all sorts of things (some of which in the past she had hated or wouldn't even try). She was now eating very close to normal size portions and had been for about 10 days. The eating didn't improve her weight and she still looked painfully thin. However she was to see the specialist nurse on Friday

17th August and was to be weighed.

She was still very tired and even with the intake of food could not do very much. What little she did achieve exhausted her and she had to sit down. She was in bed by 6 pm and didn't get up apart for going to the bathroom until 10 am the following day.

Still we did not grumble. We were better off than we were the month before. We saw the specialist nurse, but for some reason she failed to weigh Margaret, so we didn't know whether her weight had improved. She was too concerned to weigh herself on our bathroom scales, so we never knew. There was however a concern about her blood count and it was muted that there might be a need for a blood transfusion. We needed to wait until the 30th August for her next blood test to find out if it was going to be necessary.

Margaret was put back on steroids to help her eat, because as soon as she stopped taking them, her eating diminished. This brought her back to eating fairly well although not such large portions.

The 24th August was a week off from chemotherapy, much to Margaret's delight. But she was due back the following week, followed by another 2 weeks. She was then due for a CT scan to see if there was any change to the tumour. If there was then the chemotherapy would probably continue. If there wasn't any change or the tumour had become worse then Margaret was going to call it a day.

The 26th August was a particularly good day in that Margaret felt so good that she managed to do more than she had done for some time. They were only little things, but things non the less.

When we looked back over the past few months, we realised that now we were in a far better place than we had been. But we were still taking each day as it came as tomorrow could be very different.

The chemotherapy on the 31st August took place and the blood count had improved so the need for a blood transfusion had now passed.

OUT OF OUR HANDS

Unfortunately after the Friday chemotherapy session Margaret wasn't so good, which was such a shame as she was doing so well. The biggest problem she was having were her bowel movements. Although she avoided the curse of diarrhoea, the frequency of bowel movements was quite something. Even in the early hours of the morning, she was woken with an urgent need for the loo. At this time she was still managing just about to get to the toilet by herself, but it was a struggle and I was awake awaiting her return.

Margaret made a decision at this time that at the end of the next 3 week period of chemotherapy, she would wait until after her next CT scan and the appointment with the Oncologist before deciding whether to continue with the chemotherapy, assuming of course she was given the option. She was tired of the discomfort, the traveling, having needles poked into her and the concern that very soon the nurses would be unable to find a suitable vein for the cannula. Of course I was going to stand by her whatever her decision, but if it was me I wouldn't continue.

Margaret wasn't having a very good time, after all the improvement, she seemed to be slipping back. The chemotherapy session on 7th September proved to be her last visit. After waiting for an hour to be seen, we were told that the HB levels were too low for chemotherapy to take place. After some discussion with the Macmillan specialist nurse it was decided to discontinue the chemotherapy as there were only 2 more sessions. He said that at this stage missing the last two sessions would make no difference to the end result. If the chemotherapy had worked, the sessions she had already undergone would be sufficient.

Having stopped the chemotherapy, Margaret seemed to make a little improvement. Whether it was the relief of knowing that the sessions had stopped I'm not sure. From my point of view it was a relief not having to do the journey to the hospital. The CT scan was brought forward to the 19th September, with an appointment to see the Oncologist on 26th September. We were to find out if the chemotherapy had worked. What was to happen from this point on was any-ones guess. But as always we kept plodding on taking each moment as it happened.

The 19th September came and we went for the CT scan. We arrived an hour earlier than the 12.15 pm appointment time. Another rush to get there as Margaret was even slower now so to be at the hospital by 11.15 am meant leaving home at the latest 10.30 am. I still had to walk the dogs get myself ready and help Margret. Looking back I'm not sure how I managed it all. I have a job getting myself ready for an appointment now.

The reason for the early arrival was to drink 2 liters of a vile clear liquid over the period of an hour. The liquid smelt like aniseed but didn't taste anything like it. Ten minutes before she was called in for the scan, she was taken through to another room to have a cannula fitted in order that a dye could be injected into it. We waited an hour longer than expected, it was now 1.15 pm before the scan took place. The scan was only 15 minutes after a 2 hour wait. Now all we had to do was wait for the result, when we see the Oncologist on 26th September. It was out of our hands now.

Whilst waiting for the appointment Margaret wasn't too good at all. Still very tired and was now suffering from a pain in the left side of her chest. We thought she may have cracked a rib as I had to lift her because she slipped down the bed and because she had lost so much weight it would be any easy thing to do.

THE ONCOLOGIST APPOINTMENT

The meeting with the Oncologist went well. The chemotherapy had shrunk the tumour by 2 cm which in itself was great news. However the consultant pointed out that this didn't mean Margaret was getting better, just given her a little more time. I questioned why if the tumour had shrunk Margaret wasn't beginning to feel better as to me this would be the logical process. He explained that the chemotherapy treatment would still be in a her system and this was the reason she still felt so poorly. In view of that he decided that the chemotherapy would stop for 6 weeks to give Margaret time for her general health and tiredness to improve. An appointment was made for the 7th November when it was to be decided how to proceed.

Whilst we were there I mentioned the pain in Margaret's rib cage and back. The consultant checked the CT scan again to see whether there was a cause for this, but he could find nothing. He put it down to a pulled muscle but I'm afraid I wasn't convinced.

So all we could do was to continue as we were taking each day as it came. Going out if we can and staying in when my friend felt too ill. That was the last time we were to see the Oncologist although we didn't realise it at the time.

INCREASED PAIN

After the meeting with the Oncologist Margaret's pain increased. As to the exact cause we never knew, but it seemed to be in her bones, back, ribs and arms but as yet not in her legs. The pain made movement difficult and apart from getting up to wash and use the toilet she stayed in bed. This started on 30th September. The pain killers she was prescribed didn't seem to have much effect and all in all she was extremely miserable. I knew at this point that the next stage was going to be even more difficult than what we had already been through. Fortunately the 'Clexane' injections had now been stopped, because now the chemotherapy had stopped there was no need for them.

With increasing pain and her existing painkillers seeming useless, Margaret finally agreed to meet with the district nurse and case supervisor on Monday 22nd October. They recommended a change to her medication, suggesting an opiate based drug, but Margaret would have none of it. I tried to persuade her that she would feel much more comfortable, but no she would not budge. So a compromise was made by introducing a stronger version of the medication she was all ready taking 'Tramadol'. This worked some of the time, but she still had periods of pain.

THE DETERIORATION

The biggest problem we were facing was the rapid deterioration. It was very sudden. Up until this point Margaret had managed to get herself to and from the toilet unaided even during the night and was still managing to shower or bath herself with my supervision.

This had now changed. I had to take my friend to the toilet day and night and wipe her bottom as she no longer seemed capable of this. I was washing her and she was spending all of her time in bed. She was eating even less even though she was taking tablets to improve her appetite. It wasn't only the physical deterioration, her mind seemed to be failing too.

Using the remote control for the TV in the bedroom she would periodically call out that the TV had gone off. When I checked it had been switched off. I questioned her, but she would deny doing it, because she didn't realise or remember she had switched it off. I watched her and she would play with the buttons on the remote, flicking from channel to channel and complaining that the channel kept changing whilst she was watching something and then she would switch it off. She was totally unaware. I can see the funny side now, but at the time I must admit I did get a bit cross with her because I thought she was doing it deliberately. I knew then that things were going to be very difficult indeed and I hoped there was an end in sight, more for Margaret, because she would have hated being as she was if she had realised. I prayed that Great Spirit would help me through each day.

By 3rd November the deterioration was continuing. I was up two or three times in the night to take her to the toilet. Th bowels were being very active again, where it was all coming from when she wasn't eating anything, was beyond me, but there was tons of it. I thought she had finished, began to wipe her bottom and she would do some more. It was a nightmare. I was so tired, exhausted, I guess most of the time I was on auto pilot.

Margaret had the permanent shakes, a bit like the DT's, but I guess that was lack of sustenance. She was now eating even less if that was possible and every time she put anything in her mouth she retched. This included her medication. She became really crafty with this, a bit like a child a suppose. She would pretend she had swallowed it and then I would find it under her tongue or in the side of her cheek. So the painkillers
weren't even getting into her system.

Margaret wanted to die at home, but with the deterioration, lack of fluid intake, and unable to take her medication I was beginning to wonder whether this was going to be possible.

Even when she did actually swallow the tablets they only took the edge off the pain, so she was in constant discomfort and when I lifted her, I knew I was hurting her but what could I do. I was sure she had given up because when I tried to encourage her and be positive, which believe me wasn't easy, she became very agitated and shouted at me to leave her alone. The road got harder and it got harder still. I thanked Great Spirit for continuing to help me through it.

NEARING THE END

On the 8th November we had an unexpected visit from the District nurse. She came to take Margaret's blood pressure. After she had completed the task, I took her to one side out of Margaret's ear shot and explained what had been happening and how she was deteriorating. She was very understanding and arranged a whole gambit of things as she felt that what was happening was the beginning of the end. She wasn't really telling me anything I hadn't already realised but it was good in some ways to get the confirmation.

She arranged for Morphine to ease the pain during the night and for a doctor to call, otherwise when the time came Margaret would need a post mortem. Apparently even though she was under a doctor, she still needed to be seen by a G.P. which so far since the appointment on the 8th May hadn't happened. She had seen doctors and consultants at the hospital, but this didn't count, unless the person dies in the hospital.

This had all come about since the Harold Shipman case. The G.P. visit was arranged for the following Friday 16th November. I just hoped that it wasn't going to be too late. I hoped for Margaret's sake that it wasn't going to be a long drawn out affair and that the end would be quick and peaceful.

WHAT THE DOCTORS DON'T TELL YOU

By now it was the 11th November Remembrance Sunday. Margaret continued on the downward spiral at an alarming rate. What they didn't tell you and by they I mean the medical profession, is exactly what lay ahead for the dying Pancreatic Cancer Patient.

I suppose I understood why they didn't tell the patient, but I thought they should explain to the carer or family what should be expected. Some of what happened to Margaret, I managed to confirm from my internet searches. But the reality of living through this stage is something quite different.

So what is to be expected as a carer or by the family. I will be very explicit.

- Your loved one will stop eating, they will still drink small amounts, but this will eventually stop.
- Their speech will become slurred and unintelligible.
- If they wear false teeth, the teeth become too big for the mouth because of the weight loss, and keep falling out. Towards the end when the retching begins they can be no longer be tolerated in the mouth at all.
- They present similar symptoms to Alzheimer's Disease. They become confused and in my case kept calling out for their 'Mummy' who passed away some 40 years earlier.
- They become agitated and frustrated because they can no longer make themselves understood.

- *They will become incontinent, in my case it was the bowels, not realising that they needed to go to the toilet.*
- *They can no longer pee, in my case the longest period was 32 hours, I think this is due to everything starting to shut down (kidney failure)*
- *The eyes became distant and manifested an appearance of fear.*
- *They can't support themselves at all as they are so weak, because they are just skin and bone with no muscles to support them.*
- *They become almost a stranger to you as they are no longer the person you knew.*
- *I doesn't matter how many times you wash them, they smell. It was a horrible smell coming from the pores of the skin. I suppose it was the toxins trying to escape and the body dying from the inside. I guess it was the 'smell of death'.*
- *Towards the very end they will shout a 'grunting' sort of noise every few seconds and this goes on day and night.*

Coping with this stage of the illness was for me the most difficult part. I wished someone had warned me. I didn't know how anyone could still survive when every bone in their body was exposed through a thin layer of skin and their internal organs were obviously not functioning properly if at all. I prayed that it may all end soon for Margaret's sake. If she had really understood what was happening to her she would have been appalled.

MY CRISIS POINT

The weekend of the 10th and 11th November were my crisis point. Margaret having taken a dramatic turn for the worse. She was only managing to pee once in 24 hours if that and when she did go it was dark brown again. She kept asking for the toilet but when I took her and put her on the loo, she said she either didn't want to go now or just couldn't. I tried all sorts of tricks to try and get her to pee, went away and ignored her because I thought me standing watching may put her off, turning on the taps, but nothing worked.

The reverse of the coin was that she was becoming incontinent with her bowels and again there was so much of it. I was at breaking point and trying to hold up an uncooperative body that needed cleaning and changing after opening her bowels, I admit I was struggling and it's sods law that it happens at a weekend when you are unable to contact anyone. To top it all Margaret suddenly became confused with Alzheimer's Disease type symptoms. This was caused by the toxins reaching the brain.

I sat on the side of the bath with Margaret in her wheelchair and sobbed. I didn't mean to do it in front of here but I couldn't cope anymore. I just said to her

'I'm sorry I just can't do this on my own anymore, I've got to get some help, I know you didn't want that, but I just can't do it'.
I didn't think at the time she had understood because there was no response or recognition as to what I had said.

By Monday morning 12th November, I knew I had to make some phone calls. The troops arrived in force. The G.P., nurses I had them all.

I knew how bad Margaret was because she made no complaint about the G.P being there and it was the G.P that she had a very low opinion of and had missed the 'lump'. I know for sure had she been in her right mind she would have told him to get out. As it was, she mad no comment apart from 'I do know what's going on you know'.

Margaret was fitted with a catheter and a syringe pump, which administered the morphine. Incontinence sheets were placed under her so the need to try and get her to the toilet was no longer necessary. Which was just as well, because not long before they all arrived I had taken her to the bathroom using the wheelchair. I'd been getting her to the bathroom like this for some days. I'd had to move furniture about to accommodate the wheelchair , but it was easier than try to walk her. I managed to get her onto the toilet, but then when I tried to get her off she just collapsed on me. I thought she had died then.

There was nothing, no response and she had crumpled onto her knees and it was only my body stopping her. I struggled and struggled to get her back in the wheelchair. Even though she was normally so light she was a dead weight. I managed in the end, I'm not sure how. By the time I got her back to the bedroom she seemed to come back to life and getting her into bed was much easier.

THE FINAL DAY

Monday night into Tuesday morning was a restless night. Margaret grunted loudly every few seconds all evening, all through the night and into Tuesday morning. In some ways it was quite funny because periodically I would say 'Margaret shut up' and she would say 'Sorry' and then start again within seconds. But joking apart she was obviously in distress, so I contacted the nurses again on the morning of 13th November. They returned and added a sedative to the syringe pump which had the desired effect and calmed her.

Before they arrived she seemed to have a more lucid moment and said very clearly,
'I am going to die now'
I replied,
'Yes I think you are in the next couple of days'.

Then she went back into her daze.

Margaret remained very peaceful after her sedative. The Hospice nurses came with a view to coming in and helping me with washing and changing her. Shortly after their arrival, one of the nurses went to check on Margaret and realised that her breathing pattern had changed. There were no pulses on the limbs and it was assumed that the end was very near. This was around 1 pm. The nurses kindly offered to stay with me, which I accepted as I didn't really fancy being alone. However Margaret had her own ideas about when was appropriate to go and after an hour and no change, the nurses had to go as they had other patients to see.

So there I was on my own not knowing when the end would be. I sat on the bed beside her and told that the nurses had gone so it was OK to go now. I told her I was sorry if I shouted at her and got impatient at times, but it hadn't been easy for either of us. I told her it was all right to go, that me and the dogs would be fine and to stop fighting the inevitable. I know she heard me because although everything else was effectively dead, she raised an eyebrow, just like she had if she wasn't sure if what you were saying was true or not, It sort of said 'Yeah right'.

I kept popping in and out of the bedroom, telling her that it was OK to go, to stop fighting it, but it took her another 2 hours. I'd just popped out and when I went back she had passed. It was 4 pm. There was part of me that felt guilty that I wasn't with her at the moment of death, because that meant she died alone! To be honest there are times when I still do. But the other part of me was relieved that I wasn't there because I didn't want to see her die.

It's daft what you do, but I needed to make sure that she was dead before I called the doctor to certify death and it wasn't that her breathing was so shallow that it just looked that way. I put my hand under her nose to feel any breath and I put my ear to her chest, to see if I could hear a heartbeat. I tried to close her eyes, but they insisted on popping open again so I gave up on that. I let the dogs come in to the bedroom and smell Margaret, they knew there was something wrong anyway. They have never looked for her since that day.

I lit a candle and burnt some incense sticks and put on a Music for Healing CD. I prayed to Great Spirit to help Margaret pass over into the spirit world. I then telephoned the surgery and waited for the doctor to come and confirm death. I then phoned the undertaker.

The doctor came, but it wasn't the doctor that had seen Margaret the previous day. So whilst he was quite happy to confirm death and release the body, he couldn't sign the death certificate. This had to be carried out by the doctor that saw her. This happens quite often and is nothing to be concerned about. Whilst the doctor was present I asked if he could remove the catheter and syringe pump. He did do it but he wouldn't have done unless I'd asked. I'm not sure who he thought would have done it because the undertaker certainly wouldn't.

The next couple of hours are very hazy. I'm not sure if I ate or not. I do remember feeding the dogs. At 6 pm on Tuesday 13th November Margaret left home for the last time. But she did get her last wish, which was to die at home. She would be coming back in a different form as she wanted her ashes buried in the front garden. This happened very unceremoniously with just me and many tears on 1st December 2012. Where she lays is marked with three Meerkats one of her favourites from the Compare the Market .com insurance comparison site.

THE FUNERAL

Margaret wanted a civil ceremony which was duly arranged. She was cremated as was her wish on 23rd November 2012. The following is the eulogy that I read out at the service and a poem written by me.

All of you here today have known Margaret in some way. Some of you have known her for many years, others have known her for a relatively short period of time. But I'm sure you will all agree that in her own way she has impacted on your life.

Margaret first came into my life in 1987 when we began to work together. At that time I was her boss and she never let me forget it. Many a time she would say ' You're not my boss now'! In fact I think the roll was reversed as she 'bossed' me about enough.

She had a varied working life and whilst working in television, she met the rich and famous as well as traveling abroad. Later she moved into nursing and witnessed the miracle of birth. Her move from London to Kent brought her into contact with Adults with Learning Difficulties and as a Day center officer she excelled in teaching, in particular Adult Literacy.

Although many of you will know Margaret as a lively, funny person there were aspects of her personal life, especially when she was young that were often less positive and traumatic. These traumas involved both her health and the people she loved and cared for and sometimes the consequences of this made her unhappy.

Margaret's great passion in life was her garden, clever clogs that she was, could name some plants by their Latin names, unlike myself who can barely distinguish a weed from a cultivated plant. She also loved cleaning, now who in their right mind loves cleaning? She used to love standing back and admiring the sparkling bathroom sink. Quite frankly I was scared to use it, once it had been cleaned. She also loved to watch the birds on the feeders in the garden. Whilst poorly she could watch them through the window from the comfort of her bed.

Margaret has been many things to many people, most of those people are here today. To me Margaret was first and foremost my friend and it wasn't until 2002 that we realised that there was much more to our friendship. I found a letter which she wrote to me in January 2002 and this is what she said,

'It is such a great feeling to know that I am loved so much and it makes me feel very warm, safe and secure, something that I have not felt for many years. So thank you for everything. You have taught me so many things in life and I'm sure there are many more things I will learn from you. So not only do I love you so very much, I have a lot to thank you for.' She taught me many things too.

It was an honour and a privilege to know her and I know our paths will cross again.

WHAT IS DEATH

Death is just the beginning
If only you could see
No longer trapped inside my shell
My spirit soaring free.

Death is just the beginning
I don't want you to grieve
I'm in another dimension
Still close, so please believe.

Death is just the beginning
Rejoice that my spirit is free
It sores and leaps with joy and love
If only you could see.

Death is just the beginning
Of a journey yet to follow
Standing there beside you
I'll still be there tomorrow.

Ann Elizabeth Bruce 2010

A YEAR ON

It doesn't seem possible that just a year ago, I experienced what you have just read. In some ways it seems much longer and in others it doesn't feel that it was me who actually went through it with Margaret.

I thought I would be OK on my own, that I didn't need anyone to care for or love, but I was wrong. Even though I keep myself very busy, apart from when I'm on the computer either on the internet or like now writing this book, I'm on the go all the time. Walking the dogs, cleaning the house, which seems to be constant, decorating for the sake of it really. So far I've repaired and repainted the outside of the garage, painted the garden fences, removed the old tiles from both the kitchen and bathroom and replaced them. Emulsioned a bedroom because I didn't like the colour.

I have many acquaintances where I live but no friends. Everyday seems the same, I'm never quite sure what day of the week I'm on, but I have to keep going and hope that it will all change soon. I'm ready to move on, I've never been one to mope about and feel sorry for myself although sometimes that can prove difficult.

Any way enough about me. Just to say that I hope if you have gone to the trouble of purchasing and reading this book it has been helpful to you. We can achieve anything whether we think we are capable of it or not. Love is the key.

IN LOVING MEMORY OF

MARGARET

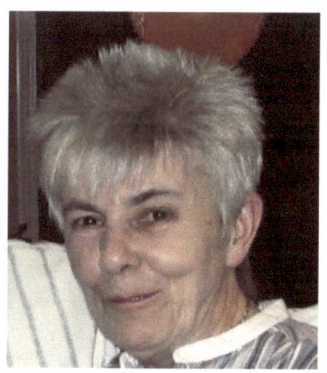

1ˢᵗ April 1945 – 13ᵗʰ November 2012